Symbolic 6
Temple Invasion

The Truth About Why You
Are Not Losing Weight!

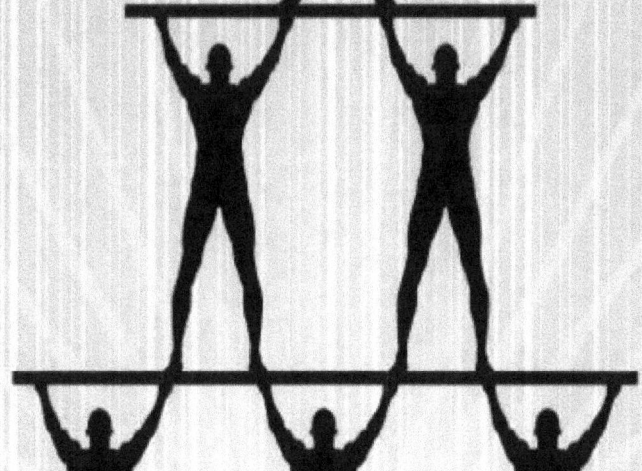

Koocie Montgomery

The Symbolic 6
Temple Invasion

The Truth About Why You Are Not Losing Weight

Published in the United States of America
ISBN: **978-1519433626**
$5.00

Table of Contents

Chapter 1
Leeks & Onions

Most often, your weight loss treasure is right under your nose! However, it's up to you whether or not you take the time or the opportunity to get rid of the junk and sift through the dirt to get to what rightfully belongs to you, and that is getting your body back.

Jesus awarded us the Holy Spirit when He ascended into heaven, even though we may not have been worthy of it at the time, but He awarded the wealth of the Holy Spirit anyway. Being healthy is your divine birthright, waiting for you to claim it. It has nothing to do with your marketing strategies, tricks or tactics—this is your "MANNA" for the journey. It's all about possessing what is already within YOU!

When the Children of Israel came out of Egypt, God provided a guide to them automatically, a cloud by day and a pillar of fire by night. Of course, it was taken for granted. Now, the guide (the Holy Spirit) will not be given to us automatically, we have to accept Him into our lives. Most people believe that there is a Holy Spirit, but negates the fact that the Holy Spirit is the most important factor and the divine connection to their successful weight loss.

Weight loss is not just about losing the weight; it's really about losing the inner pain that keeps you fat. If you would dare to trust the Holy Spirit with your eating habits, or emotional rollercoasters, He will provide you with Direction (He will lead the way), purpose (He will illuminate the purpose that He has for your life), Provision (He will provide for the vision) and He will help you pray for things or issues that are unknown to you.

As the Children of Israel journeyed through the desert, they became hungry. As usual, they complained to Moses about it—it behooves me that they were willing to go back into bondage and slavery just to fill their stomachs with fish, leeks, onion, garlic, melons and cucumbers at no cost. They did not realize that it wasn't really for free! However, Moses prayed to God, despite their vicious complaints, and God rained bread from heaven, which is commonly known as manna.

God also gave them many different ways to prepare the manna, and the Children of Israel were still not satisfied—they wanted more. They wanted meat, if God intended for them to live off of meat, He would have rained down meat instead of manna or meat in conjunction with the manna. In fact, having meat was never God's original plan for them. God's first plan was THE PROMISED LAND with MILK AND HONEY! His second plan was to feed them bread from heaven. He was trying to deal with their slave mentality, and they were focused on their next meal, oppose to their next step. My friend, they spoke of freedom and continually thought about slavery—this is definitely an indication that the price of bricks and mud was more valuable to them than the freedom to create a life of whatever they wanted.

After the Children of Israel constantly complained to Moses about meat, God gave them meat to feed their fleshly cravings. He did not give them meat for one day as He does with the daily ration of manna—He gave them meat for a whole month. While giving into the murmurs and the lust of their flesh, they overindulged by partaking too much of something that they were not supposed to have anyway. By this one act of greed, eating too much meat caused a parasitic plague that took the lives of many. As a result, they still did not get the big picture; which provides us with an opportunity to go right, where they went wrong. The wilderness experience is designed to purge you from the desire of wanting or giving in to your fleshly desires. My friend, GOD HEARS ALL MURMURS, and now is not the time to murmur about what you don't have or how fat you are, this is a time of soul searching to understand the deeper meaning of the manna that's presented in your life. Going through this phase, you will definitely have to walk by faith, and not by sight. This is where your faith will be developed, put to the test and polished. However, with **The Symbolic 6 Diet Plan**, you are required to cut back on eating meat; however, at this point, there are 2 things we need to worry about, and this is GERMS and WORMS!

Chapter 2
The Unknown

The factor of the unknown or better yet, the things that we ignore keeps us aloof about what's really happening with our bodies. I often hear people saying, "Oh no, that will never happen to me." Well, believe it or not, it's happening right now if we have never taken the time to cleanse our bodies. I have found that the things that we can't see are more powerful than the things that we can see. For example, we can't see germs, but they have the power to kill us. We can't see most parasites, and here again they will kill us if they are not properly controlled. Although we proclaim to be a germaphobic nation; but somehow we miss the bandwagon on parasites. For some odd reason, we think that this is only an epidemic in 3rd World Countries; as a result, sickness and disease is running rampant among us here in the Land of the

Free—as the Bible states, "My people parish for the lack of knowledge."

The most significant part of our **Symbolic 6 Diet Plan** is the Detoxification phase, and we make that as a prerequisite for a reason. Where there's a longing, we must take into account the seeds that we have planted over the years. When we take into account what we are giving, then we are better able to understand what we are receiving. My friend, everything, and I mean everything we do, say, think, eat and drink becomes a SEED! And, it is up to us to determine whether or not our seeds will become positively or negatively planted, discarded, or held on to.

Life has a way of granting us the conditions in which we subconsciously choose. When given a little time, the seed that we plant can and will produce after its own kind, regardless of when, what, how, where and why it's planted. But, what about the seeds that remain unplanted? Great question, "NO HARVEST!" There are some seeds that we need to plant and there are some that we should not plant.

Your lifeline is in the seeds that you are planting in your body mentally, physically, emotionally, and spiritually. Don't think for a minute that you are able to supersede the laws of the land, "SEED, TIME and HARVEST." If we are eating badly, with time the harvest will come; and for that reason, it is imperative that we detox our body. If our body is full of toxins, it is definitely harder to lose weight, because our body begins to fight us back. The Symbolic 6 Temple Invasion deals with 2 types of Toxins:

1. Toxins from Foods
2. Toxins from a Parasitic Infestation

Both types of toxins are bad for our bodies, and need to be dealt with appropriately, if not we will get sick, gain weight, or have hormonal imbalances that causes major health issues.

Chapter 3
Enemies Within

It is a common misconception that parasites can be prevented by washing our fruits and vegetables, and cooking our meat well. However, what they don't tell us is that does not always do the trick—parasites are smarter than we are, and they know how to hide themselves very well. Remember, parasites do not multiply like bacteria or mold, in order for them to thrive and survive, they need a host (Human or Animal); therefore, they will do anything to leave a legacy of their lineage. Parasites, like Cyclospora, Cryptosporidium, and Giardia, are all resistant to our standard level of chlorine found in regular drinking water and swimming pools. As a matter of fact, some parasites can survive through filtered or boiled water depending upon the appropriate condition.

Most contamination or transmission takes place through water, food, and bathrooms in addition to the germs that are already taking up residence. We cannot get away from the critters; we can only prepare ourselves with the appropriate tools to combat them.

How do we know if we have a parasitic infestation in our body that's causing problems? Let's start with stomach problem such as:

- Abdominal Pain
- Bloating
- Bloody in Stool
- Burning in the Stomach
- Chronic Constipation
- Diarrhea
- Digestive Problems
- Excessive Early Bowel Movements
- Excessive Gas
- Explosive bowel movements
- Hemorrhoids
- Leaky Gut
- Mucus in the Stools
- Nausea

The toxic overloads and overworks the organs while attacking the central nervous system causing:

- Chronic Fatigue Syndrome
- Excessive Weakness
- Lethargy

- Low Energy

When tissue becomes inflamed from the toxins, the body's white blood cells increase to defend the body. This reaction causes skin rashes and food allergies to appear, as well as the following symptoms:

- Allergic Reactions to Food
- Allergies
- Brittle Hair
- Crawling Sensation under the Skin
- Ulcers
- Dry Hair
- Dry Skin
- Hair Loss
- Hives
- Itchy Anus
- Itchy Nose
- Itchy Skin
- Lesions
- Rashes
- Sores
- Swelling
- Eczema

These little critters that lurk from within can and will contribute to our mental instability issues causing:

- Anxiety
- Depression
- Forgetfulness
- Mood Swings
- Nervousness
- Restlessness
- Slow Reflexes
- Unclear Thinking

When the body is at rest, the toxic invasion of parasites takes over the body causing:

- Bed Wetting
- Disturbed Sleep
- Drooling While Asleep
- Insomnia
- Seizures
- Sudden Jilts while sleeping
- Teeth Grinding

To say the least, they also cause appetite, malnutrition, and weight disorders such as:

- Constantly Feeling Hungry
- Inability to Gain Weight
- Lose Weight

- Loss of Appetite
- Obesity
- Weight Gain Even When Being Malnourished

However these little rug rats can travel to almost all soft tissue, taking over the joints and muscle. Once that is done, they begin to cause cysts and inflammation build up, which gets commonly mistaken as arthritis and muscle pain. And when they pool together, they cause:

- Arthritic Pains
- Back Pain
- Fast Heartbeat
- Heart Pain
- Joint Pain
- Muscle Cramping
- Muscle Pain
- Numbness of the Hands and/or Feet
- Pain in the Navel
- Shoulder Pain

These blood suckers take all the good vitamins, including iron; therefore, causing one to become:

- Diabetic
- Severely Anemic

Not only that, they cause one to have a weakened immune system causing:

- Cysts & Fibroids
- Erectile Dysfunction
- Menstrual Problems
- PMS
- Prostate Problems
- Urinary Tract Infections
- Water Retention
- Yeast Infections

This parasitic moocher also causes:

- Bad Breath
- Body Odor
- Excessive Saliva
- Fever
- Peritonitis
- Poor Immune Response
- Respiratory Problems
- Unclear Vision

As we can see, parasites are contributing to most of our health issues, but are not diagnosed as such. As most of us don't want to talk about this issue; but, if our bodies are becoming more infected by these microscopic intruders, we must do something about it. Now, it's up to us to take charge of our health and not allow something that we cannot see, cause us to lose ourselves outwardly. Doctors are not going to tell us that parasites are a major cause of our diseases, weight gain, fatigue, brain fogs, vision problems, and much more—this will cut off their residual income. Or, better yet, they will not be able to overload us with habit forming prescriptions to keep us legally hooked on drugs. There is a reason why the Drug Stores are on every corner; however, this is not designed for one to ignore medical attention or to stop taking their prescription medication, this is designed to bring awareness to what's really taking place within **The Temple of the Holy Spirit**.

For this parasitic reason, The **Symbolic 6 Detox** is a prerequisite before embarking upon this weight loss plan. In order to effectively maximize this program, order your Detox at www.Symbolic6.com. Furthermore, if we deworm our pets, why are we not deworming ourselves? The eggs are all around us, and that is why 73% of the population today is unawaringly infected. This is an epidemic that is directly linked to our obesity, sicknesses, and diseases.

Today, choose your seeds carefully, as you discard the negative seeds that are intentionally or unintentionally causing havoc in your body to ensure that you are ready for the real Manna.

Chapter 4

Temple Invasion

We must learn how to eat healthy to keep the infestation of these little body snatchers down; although, eating out is nice at times, but we must ask ourselves if it is healthy for us. There are a lot of things that we are not being told regarding the things that we are consuming daily, because if we knew the truth—a lot of Stores, Restaurants, Doctor's offices, and Drug Stores would go out of business.

It may be a shock to discover that parasites play a critical role in our lives, and have a vital capacity on earth; therefore we are exposed to them each day with or without our consent. In order to enhance and look after our wellbeing, it is vital to understand their purpose, and how to prevent them from infecting or taking over our bodies. God has designed parasites to have an imperative function on earth; and that is to feast upon rotting, decaying matter, until it comes back to the earth creating soil that feeds the plants, animals and all of mankind. Parasites are designed to gravitate toward the weak, mutating, and dying cells to further break them down. In so many words, the weaker vessel becomes infected to make room for healthier and livelier vessels; which is applicable to human life, animal life, plant life, or better yet, every living thing on the face of this earth. According to Genesis 3:19 it says clearly, "By the sweat of your face You will eat bread, Till you return to the ground, Because from it you were taken; For you are dust, And to dust you shall return." However, we do not want to go back to the dust before our time—Yes, Adam and Eve disobeyed God in the Garden of Eden and reaped the punishment of death to all mankind, but God also granted us the wisdom to prolong our life as well.

We can say that it's gross all that we want, but for those who are ignorant to the reality of parasitic infestations are really not the ones who should be judging whether or not parasites are really gross. Instead, they should learn as much as possible to take the proper precautions to protect themselves as well as others. If we saw a parasite, most often we would not know that it's a parasite. Although, most parasites are microscopic in nature; however, some parasites look like fat deposits, eggs, or mucus that's passed along in our feces, saliva, and other bodily fluids.

When we don't get the adamant amount of water, air, sleep, exercise, or nutrients, our bodies become susceptible to:

1. Overeating
2. Shamefulness
3. Needy in a Relationship
4. Subjective to Peer Pressure
5. Mentally Deprived
6. Laziness or Slothfulness
7. Fearful
8. Emotional Stress
9. Greed
10. Lack of Determination
11. Guilt
12. Loneliness
13. Depression

Now, the key is that parasites love, and prey on those who are dealing with such issues. That becomes their playground to run rampant and take control without being detected as a parasitic invasion. And, when we go to the Doctor, they will treat the symptoms, and not the cause; therefore, creating a win-win situation for the Doctor, the Drug Store, the Pharmaceutical Company, and the critter from within. In my opinion, that's a lifetime membership for them to feed, because with medication, it helps in one area and breaks down another with toxins. The side-effects are written on the bottle, and we still become ignorant to the fact that there's a deeper problem that needs to be resolved, such as taking the bull by the horn and become HEALTHY! Make no mistake about it, medication is good for those who need it, but most often, we are taking medication for symptoms caused by parasites, because our Doctors today are trained to deal with the symptoms and not the causes.

Our bodies will naturally heal itself if one would take the time out to learn what to put in our bodies, how to detox our bodies, and what types of food to stay away from or limit. A diet rich in raw garlic, pumpkin seeds, carrots, beets, pineapples, papaya seeds and pomegranates can help control and kill parasites that invades our body trying to claim us as a host. Once they are dead, we must flush them out of our body by keeping our system regular by going to the bathroom. Fiber is good; however, we have the **Symbolic 6 Cleansing Tea** that will assist that process. God forbid if we are not going to the bathroom—rest assured that is a nesting place for these little creatures to invade, take-over, and migrate to different areas of our bodies creating the silent killer from within.

Chapter 5

The Silent Killer

This silent killer is one of our best kept secrets. Internal parasites cause extensive damage to our bodies without us realizing what's going on until it is too late. They rob us of our valuable nutrients; they cause gastrointestinal irritations, heartburns, intestinal ruptures, intestinal blockages, and death, to say the least. They are passed from animal to people, from people to animal, and from plants to people or animal, from animal or people back to the soil, then to the plant, and then from the plant back to people or animals. What a cycle, but it is indeed the cycle of life, and if we desire not to go back to the soil before our time, we must become cognizant of what we are putting in our bodies—just because it tastes good, does not mean that it is good for us.

When I say it's a silent killer, I mean it. Doctors proclaim that they do not know what causes cancer, fibroids, fibromyalgia, PMS, Alzheimer's, and a few other diseases; however, I am stating that it's caused by a parasitic Invasion of our Temple. An infestation can be recognized by the eyes being watery, red, or having blurry vision. The skin will have rashes, pimples, eczema, blotches, white heads, or acne. The scalp will have dandruff, bumps, bald spots, or itchiness. The gums will be red, swollen, receding, bleeding, or bad breath coming out of the nostrils and one's breath is always bad. The skin will have a foul odor or a constant smell of musk. The belly will swell after eating, foods will sour on the stomach quickly, one will feel constipated after eating, or one will have a resistance to eating vegetables. The feet will have athlete's feet, jock itch, dark or thick toe nails, or an overgrowth of skin. The host will be commonly diagnosed with anemia, diabetes, heart problems, hypertension, lupus, ADHD, bipolar disorder, etc. They will also battle with anger, emotional instability, depression, erratic behavior, moodiness, etc.; therefore causing self-destructive behavior.

Do parasites have the ability to control the mind? Absolutely! They infect the brain with their mind control toxins that will cause one to crave foods that they wouldn't normally eat, it would cause one to behave in a way that's abnormal, it would cause one to engage in suicidal behavior, or participate in activities that would put them at more of a risk of unawaringly spreading the eggs. The most infected individuals will engage in unprotected sex, they may have multiple sex partners, they may love kissing, they may have a drug or prescription pill addiction, or they will crave unhealthy foods that will contribute to the overgrowth of these creatures. In all actuality we become a zombie for the parasites, it will feel as if one is walking dead among the living—clinging to life one day at a time.

If we want to rid ourselves of these unwanted visitors, we must cleanse the whole household. Unfortunately, a parasite cleansing is not as effective without everyone in the household doing the cleansing together. It is a great possibility that the individual who completed the cleansing can become reinfected when kissing an infected individual, eating after an infected individual, after having sex with an infected individual, or sharing the same bathroom with an infected individual.

People may say that one is paranoid, or they may have OCD (Obsessive Compulsive Disorder) when taking the extra precautions, but it is important to cleanse the body and our environment daily. Parasites are easily transmitted microscopically from:

- The colon
- Sex Organ
- The mouth
- Unclean hands
- Unwashed fresh fruits or vegetables
- Uncooked Meat
- Pets

In order to prevent the spreading of these hijackers, we must keep our bed linens clean, wear clean underwear, and wear clean clothes. We must also disinfect the toilet seats, bathtubs, sinks, and door handles daily. And keep our hands washed after using the restroom, when handling food, and before meals.

Chapter 6

Kick the Habit

Parasites contribute to obesity by compelling one to eat more of what they like, and what will keep the fat cells coming while they invade and get fat off of the red blood cells and the nutrients from the body; therefore, leaving an individual fat, malnourished, and depressed.

Carbohydrates such as potatoes, corn, rice, pasta, bread, and most processed foods convert into sugar, which feeds them. The more carbs we crave, the more they grow and multiply and it becomes a perfect recipe for obesity, anemia, and diabetes in overweight people.

I personally consider them the Parasite Pimps, they will do anything to become fruitful and multiply, especially the hookworms, pinworms and tapeworms, as well as the single-celled organisms like giardia, H. pyloria and candida albicans. They will spike our cravings out of nowhere, all of a sudden we crave ice cream, pastries, meat, fried foods, junk foods, alcohol, cigarettes, or sex, out of the blue. Where did the craving come from? Why did we not get a craving for vegetables, or nuts? These little Pimps create a voice of reason from within; therefore, we begin to justify our cravings in order to give in to them. Or, better yet, to keep those little Pimps from getting fussy; nevertheless, if we want to become better at controlling ourselves, we need to learn how to kick the habit.

In order to embrace **The Symbolic 6 Diet Plan**, we need to pay attention to what's going on within us as well as around us. Our path of mastery is determined by our ability to reach beyond our self-imposed limitations to assume responsibility for our actions, reactions and the lack thereof regarding our eating habits, and how we are taking care of our bodies.

Most often, it is easier to blame someone else or make excuses for our weight problem, but guess what? It doesn't solve anything. If we take a moment to look back over our lives, we will find that the issues that we are having right now, are the issues that we did not pray about, the issues that we did not seek God about, or the issues that we did not exercise the wisdom that was available to us at that time. Therefore, shifting the blame has become easier, or better yet, emotionally comforting than to take responsibility for our actions, reactions, or the lack thereof.

If our past could speak, what would it say? If our present could speak, what would it say? If our future could speak, what would it say? These are some questions that we must ask ourselves when dealing with our weight loss battle or kicking our bad habits. We cannot be clueless, or careless about what we want, what we do, what we say, or what we become. We are held accountable for our actions, reactions, or the lack thereof when it comes down to our Spiritual Walk with God, and the prayers that are going to keep us on track   Now getting down to the nitty gritty, there are a few habits that we need to kick in order to succeed on this program:

1. No sodas, not even diet sodas
2. Stay hydrated with water, minimum 8 cups a day
3. No artificial flavors
4. No processed meats
5. No packaged meals
6. Watch out for the hidden sugars
7. Only eat out of a saucer plate. If that's not possible, eat only half of your meal and save the rest for later.
8. Fresh fruit only, no canned fruits or vegetables.
9. Choose your meal or the dessert when eating; you cannot have both in the same meal.
10. Limit television, food commercial will invoke food cravings

Adhering to **The Symbolic 6 Diet Plan** is not about strict dietary confinements, staying unreasonably thin, or denying yourself of the foods you adore. It's about feeling awesome, having more vitality, enhancing your lifestyle, and balancing out your state of mind to learn how and what to eat at the appropriate times. **Symbolic**

6's ultimate goal is to help individuals to utilize straightforward weight loss tips that slice through the perplexities of losing weight and keeping it off. Therefore, offering solid eating routines that is as useful for your brain as it is for your body.

So, when you eat off plan, don't say the devil made you do it, simply say, "Your parasite made you do it!"

Get your Temple Detox at: www.Symbolic6.com

Koocie Montgomery

Order at www.Symbolic6.com

Available Products

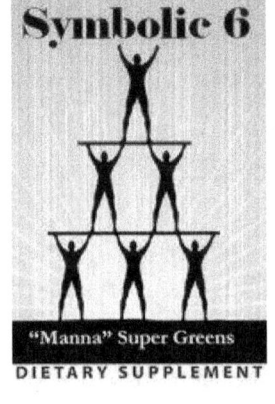
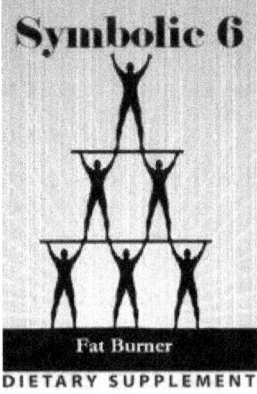
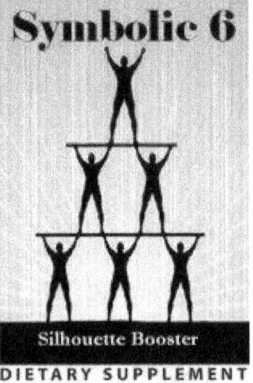

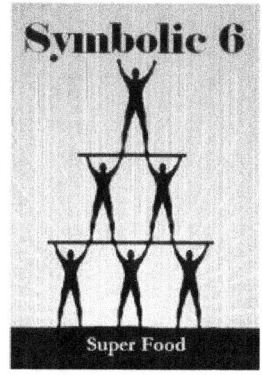

Super Food

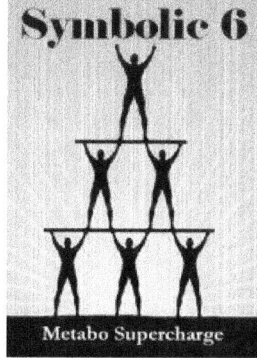

Metabo Supercharge

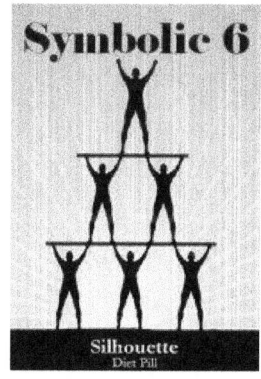

Silhouette
Diet Pill

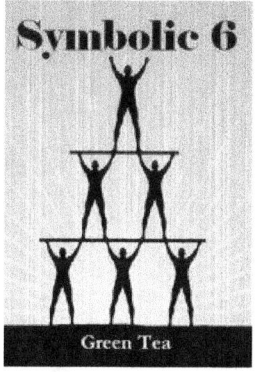

Green Tea

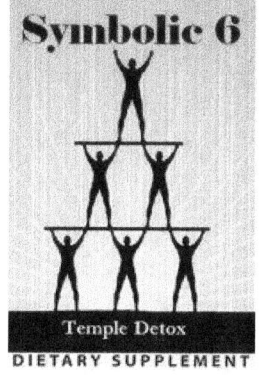

Temple Detox
DIETARY SUPPLEMENT

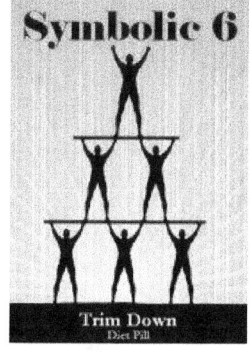

Trim Down
Diet Pill